My Lean and Green Specialties

Affordable and Creative Recipes for your Lean
and Green Diet

Carmen Bellisario

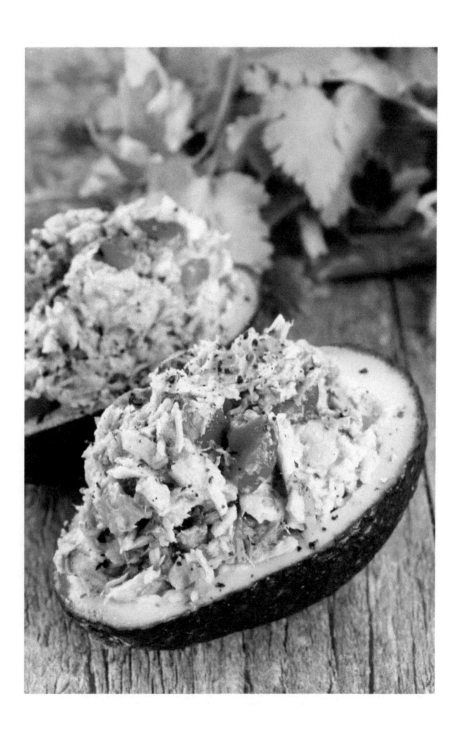

TABLE OF CONTENTS

Lemony Trout

Servings: 4

Preparation time: 15 minutes

Cooking time: 25 minutes

Ingredients:

- 2 (1½-pound) wild-caught trout, gutted and cleaned
- Salt and ground black pepper, as required
- 1 lemon, sliced
- 2 tablespoons of fresh dill, minced
- 2 tablespoon of butter, melted
- 2 tablespoons of fresh lemon juice

Instructions:

1. Preheat the oven to 475 degrees F.
2. Arrange a wire rack onto a foil-lined baking sheet.
3. Sprinkle the trout with salt and black pepper from inside and out of doors generously.
4. Fill the cavity of every fish with lemon slices and dill.
5. Place the trout onto the prepared baking sheet and drizzle with the melted butter and lemon juice.

6. Bake for about 25 minutes.

7. Remove the baking sheet from oven and transfer the trout onto a serving platter.

1. 8 Serve hot.

Tuna Stuffed Avocado

Servings: 2

Preparation time: 15 minutes

Ingredients:

- 1 large avocado, halved and pitted
- 1 tablespoon of onion, chopped finely
- 2 tablespoons of fresh lemon juice
- 5 ounces of cooked tuna, chopped
- Salt and ground black pepper, as required

Instructions:

1. With a spoon, scoop out the flesh from the centre of every avocado half and transfer into a bowl.
2. Add the onion and juice and mash until well combined.
3. Add tuna, salt and black pepper and stir to mix.
4. Divide the tuna mixture into both avocado halves evenly and serve immediately.

Fish & Spinach Curry

Servings: 4

Preparation time: 15 minutes

Cooking time: 15 minutes

Ingredients:

- 1 tablespoon of coconut oil
- 1 small yellow onion, chopped
- 2 garlic cloves, minced
- 1 teaspoon of fresh ginger, minced
- 1 large tomato, peeled and chopped
- 1 tablespoon of curry powder
- ¼ cup of water
- 1¼ cups of unsweetened coconut milk
- 1-pound of skinless grouper fillets, cubed into 2-inch size
- ¾ pound of fresh spinach, chopped
- Salt, as required
- 2 tablespoons of fresh parsley, chopped

Instructions:

1. In a large wok, melt the coconut oil over medium heat and sauté the onion, garlic and ginger for about 5 minutes.
2. Add the tomatoes and curry powder and cook for about 2-3 minutes, crushing with the rear of the spoon.
3. Add the water and coconut milk and bring to a mild boil.
4. Stir in grouper pieces and spinach and cook for about 4-5 minutes.
5. Stir in the salt and parsley and serve hot.

Crab Cakes

Servings: 4

Preparation time: 15 minutes

Cooking time: 28 minutes

Ingredients:

For Crab Cakes:

- 2 tablespoons of olive oil, divided
- ½ cup of onion, chopped finely
- 3 tablespoons of blanched almond flour
- ¼ cup of egg whites
- 2 tablespoons of mayonnaise
- 1 tablespoon of dried parsley, crushed
- 1 teaspoon of yellow mustard
- 1 teaspoon of Worcestershire sauce
- 1 tablespoon of Old Bay seasoning
- Salt and ground black pepper, to taste
- 1-pound lump crabmeat, drained

For Salad:

- 5 cups of fresh baby arugula

- 2 tomatoes, chopped
- 2 tablespoons of olive oil
- Salt and ground black pepper, to taste

Instructions:

1. For crab cakes: Heat 2 teaspoons of olive oil in a wok over medium heat and sauté onion for about 8-10 minutes.
2. Remove the frying pan from heat and put aside to chill slightly.
3. Place cooked onion and remaining Ingredients apart from crabmeat in a bowl and blend until well combined.
4. Add the crabmeat and gently, stir to mix.
5. Make 8 equal-sized patties from the mixture.
6. Arrange the patties onto a foil-lined tray and refrigerate for about 30 minutes.
7. In a large frying pan, heat remaining oil over medium-low heat and cook patties in 2 batches for about 3-4 minutes per side or until desired doneness.
8. For Salad: In a bowl, add all Ingredients, and toss to coat well.
9. Divide salad onto serving plates and to every with 2 patties.
10. Serve immediately.

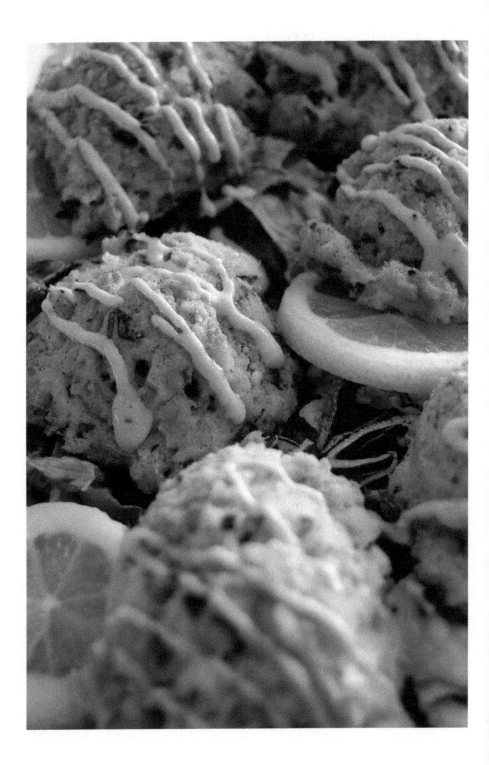

Shrimp Lettuce Wraps

Servings: 4

Preparation time: 15 minutes

Cooking time: 25 minutes

Ingredients:

- 1 teaspoon of extra-virgin olive oil
- 1 garlic clove, minced
- 1½ pounds shrimp, peeled, deveined and chopped
- Salt, as required
- 8 large lettuce leaves
- 1 tablespoon of fresh chives, minced

Instructions:

1. In a large sauté pan, heat the vegetable oil over medium heat and sauté garlic for about 1 minute.
2. Add the shrimp and cook for about 3-4 minutes.
3. Remove from heat and put aside to chill slightly.
4. 4 Arrange lettuce leaves onto serving plates.
5. Divide the shrimp over the leaves evenly.
6. Garnish with chives and serve immediately.

Shrimp Kabobs

Servings: 3

Preparation time: 15 minutes

Cooking time: 8 minutes

Ingredients:

- ¼ cup of olive oil
- 2 tablespoons of fresh lime juice
- ½ chipotle pepper in adobo sauce, seeded and minced
- 1 garlic cloves, minced
- 1½ teaspoon of powdered Erythritol
- ½ teaspoon of red chili powder
- ½ teaspoon of paprika
- ¼ teaspoon of ground cumin
- Salt and ground black pepper, as required
- 1-pound medium raw shrimp, peeled and deveined
- 5 cups of fresh salad greens

Instructions:

1. In a bowl, add all the Ingredients except the shrimp and greens and blend well.

2. Add the shrimp and coat with the herb mixture generously.
3. Refrigerate to marinate for at least 30 minutes.
4. Preheat the grill to medium-high heat.
5. Grease the grill grate.
6. Thread the shrimp onto the re-soaked wooden skewers.
7. Place the skewers onto the grill and cook for about 3-4 minutes per side.
8. Remove from the grill and place onto a platter for about 5 minutes before serving.

Shrimp with Zucchini Noodles

Servings: 4

Preparation time: 20 minutes

Cooking time: 8 minutes

Ingredients:

- 2 tablespoons of olive oil
- 1 garlic clove, minced
- ¼ teaspoon of red pepper flakes, crushed
- 1-pound shrimp, peeled and deveined
- Salt and ground black pepper, as required
- 1/3 cup of low-sodium chicken broth
- 2 medium zucchinis, spiralized with a blade
- 1 cup of cherry tomatoes, quartered

Instructions:

1. In a large non-stick skillet, heat the vegetable oil over medium heat and sauté garlic and red pepper flakes for about 1 minute.
2. Add the shrimp, salt and black pepper and cook for about 1 minute per side.

3. Add the broth and zucchini noodles and cook for about 3-4 minutes.
4. Stir in the tomato quarters and take away from the heat.
5. Serve hot.

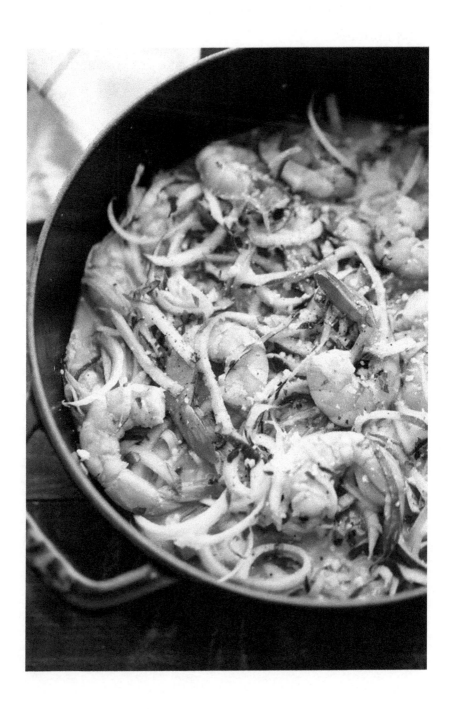

Shrimp with Spinach

Servings: 4

Preparation time: 15 minutes

Cooking time: 9 minutes

Ingredients:

- 3 tablespoons of extra-virgin olive oil
- 1-pound medium shrimp, peeled and deveined
- 1 medium onion, chopped
- 2 garlic cloves, chopped finely
- 1 fresh red chili, sliced
- 1-pound fresh spinach, chopped
- ¼ cup of low-sodium chicken broth

Instructions:

1. In a large non-stick skillet, heat 1 tablespoon of the oil over medium-high heat and cook the shrimp for about 2 minutes per side.
2. With a slotted spoon, transfer the shrimp onto a plate.

3. In the same skillet, heat the remaining 2 tablespoons of oil over medium heat and sauté the garlic and red chili for about 1 minute.
4. Add the spinach and broth and cook for about 2-3 minutes, stirring occasionally.
5. Stir in the cooked shrimp and cook for about 1 minute.
6. Serve hot.

Shrimp with Broccoli & Carrot

Servings: 5

Preparation time: 15 minutes

Cooking time: 8 minutes

Ingredients:

For Sauce:

- 1 tablespoon of fresh ginger, grated
- 2 garlic cloves, minced
- 3 tablespoons of low-sodium soy sauce
- 1 tablespoon of balsamic vinegar
- 1 teaspoon of Erythritol
- ¼ teaspoon of red pepper flakes, crushed

For Shrimp Mixture:

- 3 tablespoons of olive oil
- 1½ pounds of medium shrimp, peeled and deveined
- 12 ounces of broccoli florets
- 8 ounces of, carrot, peeled and sliced

Instructions:

1. For sauce: In a bowl, place all the Ingredients and beat until well combined. Set aside.
2. In a large wok, heat oil over medium-high heat and cook the shrimp for about 2 minutes, stirring occasionally.
3. Add the broccoli and carrot and cook about 3-4 minutes, stirring frequently.
4. Stir in the sauce mixture and cook for about 1-2 minutes.
5. Serve immediately.

Shrimp, Spinach & Tomato Casserole

Servings: 6

Preparation time: 15 minutes

Cooking time: 25 minutes

Ingredients:

- 2 tablespoons of extra-virgin olive oil
- 1 tablespoon of garlic, minced
- 1½ pounds large shrimp, peeled and deveined
- ¾ teaspoon of dried oregano, crushed
- ½ teaspoon of red pepper flakes, crushed
- ¼ cup of fresh spinach, chopped finely
- ¾ cup of low-sodium chicken broth
- 1 tablespoon of fresh lemon juice
- 2 cups of tomatoes, chopped
- 4 ounces of feta cheese, crumbled

Instructions:

1. Preheat your oven to 350 degrees F.

2. In a large skillet, heat the oil over medium-high heat and sauté the garlic for about 1 minute.
3. Add the shrimp, oregano and red pepper flakes and cook for about 4-5 minutes.
4. Stir in the spinach and salt and immediately remove from the heat.
5. Transfer the shrimp mixture into a casserole dish and spread in a good layer.
6. In the same skillet, add the broth and juice over medium heat and simmer for about 3-5 minutes or until reduces to half.
7. Stir in the tomatoes and cook for about 2-3 minutes.
8. Remove from the heat and place the tomato mixture over shrimp mixture evenly.
9. Top with feta cheese evenly.
10. Bake for about 15-20 minutes or until the top becomes golden brown.
11. Serve hot.

Prawns with Bell Pepper

Servings: 4

Preparation time: 20 minutes

Cooking time: 8 minutes

Ingredients:

- 2 tablespoons of olive oil
- 4 garlic cloves, minced
- 1 fresh red chili, sliced
- 1-pound prawns, peeled and deveined
- ½ cup of green bell pepper, seeded and julienned
- ½ cup of yellow bell pepper, seeded and julienned
- ½ cup of red bell pepper, seeded and julienned
- ½ cup of orange bell pepper, seeded and julienned
- ½ cup of white onion, sliced thinly
- ¼ cup of low-sodium chicken broth
- Salt and ground black pepper, as required

Instructions:

1. In a large non-stick skillet, heat olive oil over medium heat and sauté the garlic and red chili for about 2 minutes.
2. Add the prawn, bell peppers, onion and black pepper and fry for about 5 minutes.
3. Stir in the broth and cook for about 1 minute.
4. Serve hot.

Prawns with Broccoli

Servings: 4

Preparation time: 20 minutes

Cooking time: 10 minutes

Ingredients:

- 2 tablespoons of olive oil, divided
- 1-pound large prawns, peeled and deveined
- ½ of onion, chopped
- 3 garlic cloves, minced
- 3 cups of broccoli floret
- 2 tablespoons of low-sodium soy sauce
- Freshly ground black pepper, as required
- 2 tablespoons of fresh parsley, chopped

Instructions:

1. In a large non-stick skillet, heat 1 tablespoon of olive oil over medium heat and fry the prawns for about 1 minute per side.
2. With a slotted spoon, transfer the prawns onto a plate.

3. In the same skillet, heat the remaining oil over medium heat and sauté the onion and garlic for about 23 minutes.

4. Add the broccoli, soy sauce and black pepper and fry for about 2-3 minutes.

5. Stir in the cooked prawns and fry for about 1-2 minutes.

6. Serve hot.

Prawns with Asparagus

Servings: 4

Preparation time: 15 minutes

Cooking time: 13 minutes

Ingredients:

- 3 tablespoons of extra-virgin olive oil
- 1-pound of prawns, peeled and deveined
- 1-pound of asparagus, trimmed
- Salt and ground black pepper, as required
- 1 teaspoon of garlic, minced
- 1 teaspoon of fresh ginger, minced
- 1 tablespoon of low-sodium soy sauce
- 2 tablespoons of lemon juice

Instructions:

1. In a wok, heat 2 tablespoons of oil over medium-high heat and cook the prawns with salt and black pepper for about 3-4 minutes.
2. With a slotted spoon, transfer the prawns into a bowl. Set aside.

3. In the same wok, heat the remaining 1 tablespoon of oil over medium-high heat and cook the asparagus, ginger, garlic, salt and black pepper for about 6-8 minutes, stirring frequently.
4. Stir in the prawns and soy and cook for about 1 minute.
5. Stir in the juice and take away from the heat.
6. Serve hot.

Prawns with Kale

Servings: 4

Preparation time: 15 minutes

Cooking time: 20 minutes

Ingredients:

- 1-pound prawns, peeled and deveined
- Salt, as required
- 3 tablespoons of extra-virgin olive oil, divided
- 1 red onion, chopped finely
- 1 fresh red chili, sliced
- 1-pound fresh kale, tough ribs removed and chopped
- 3 tablespoons of low-sodium soy sauce
- 3 tablespoons of fresh orange juice
- 1 tablespoon of orange zest, grated finely
- ½ teaspoon of red pepper flakes, crushed
- Ground black pepper, as required

Instructions:

1. Season the prawns with a little salt.

2. In a large non-stick sauté pan, heat 2 tablespoons of olive oil over high heat and stir-fry the prawns for about 2-3 minutes.

3. With a slotted spoon, transfer the prawns onto a plate.

4. In the same sauté pan, heat the remaining oil over medium heat and sauté the onion for about 4-5 minutes.

5. Add the kale and stir-fry for about 2-3 minutes.

6. With a lid, cover the pan and cook for about 2 minutes.

7. Add the soy sauce, orange juice, zest, red pepper flakes and black pepper and stir to mix well.

8. Stir in the cooked prawns and cook for about 2-3 minutes.

9. Serve hot.

Scallops with Broccoli

Servings: 2

Preparation time: 15 minutes

Cooking time: 9 minutes

Ingredients:

- 2 tablespoons of olive oil
- 1 cup of broccoli, cut into small pieces
- 1 garlic clove, crushed
- ½ pound scallops
- 1 teaspoon of fresh lemon juice Salt, as required

Instructions:

1. In a large skillet, heat the oil over medium heat and cook the broccoli and garlic for about 3-4 minutes, stirring occasionally.
2. Add in the scallops and cook for about 3-4 minutes, flipping occasionally.
3. Stir in the juice and take away from the heat.
4. Serve hot.

Scallops with Asparagus

Servings: 5

Preparation time: 15 minutes

Cooking time: 10 minutes

Ingredients:

- 2 tablespoons of olive oil
- ¼ cup of yellow onion, chopped
- 2 garlic cloves, minced
- 2 tablespoons of fresh rosemary, minced
- 1-pound fresh asparagus, trimmed and cut into 1-inch pieces
- 2 teaspoons of fresh lemon zest, grated
- 1½ pounds baby scallops
- Salt and ground black pepper, as required
- 2 tablespoons of fresh lemon juice

Instructions:

1. In a large skillet, heat the oil over medium-high heat and sauté the onion for about 2 minutes.

2. Add the garlic and rosemary and sauté for about 1 minute.

3. Add the asparagus and lemon peel and cook for about 1-2 minutes.

4. Add the scallops and stir to mix.

5. Immediately reduce the heat to medium and cook, covered for about 4-5 minutes, stirring occasionally.

6. Stir in lemon juice, salt and black pepper and take away from the heat.

7. Serve hot.

Scallops with Spinach

Servings: 5

Preparation time: 15 minutes

Cooking time: 21 minutes

Ingredients:

- 1 tablespoon of olive oil
- 1½ pounds jumbo sea scallops
- Salt and ground black pepper, as required
- 1 cup of onion, chopped
- 6 garlic cloves, minced
- 14 ounces of fresh baby spinach

Instructions:

1. In a large non-stick skillet, heat the oil over medium-high heat and cook the scallops with salt and black pepper for about 5 minutes, turning once after 2½ minutes.
2. Transfer the scallops into another bowl and canopy them with a bit of foil to stay warm.
3. In the same skillet, add onion and garlic over medium heat and sauté the onion and garlic for about 3 minutes.

4. Add the spinach and cook for about 2-3 minutes.
5. Season with salt and black pepper and take away from the heat.
6. Divide the spinach onto serving plates.
7. Top with scallops and serve immediately.

Shrimp & Scallops with Veggies

Servings: 5

Preparation time: 20 minutes

Cooking time: 11 minutes

Ingredients:

- 3 tablespoons of olive oil, divided
- 1-pound of fresh asparagus, cut into 2-inch pieces
- 2 red bell peppers, seeded and chopped
- ¾ pound of medium raw shrimp, peeled and deveined
- ¾ pound of raw scallops
- 1 tablespoon of dried parsley ½ teaspoon of garlic, minced
- Salt and freshly ground black pepper, to taste

Instructions:

1. In a large skillet, heat 1 tablespoon of oil over medium heat and stir-fry the asparagus and bell peppers for about 4-5 minutes.
2. With a slotted spoon, transfer the vegetables onto a plate.

3. In the same skillet, heat the remaining oil over medium heat and stir-fry shrimp and scallops for about 2 minutes.

4. Stir in the parsley, garlic, salt, and black pepper, and cook for about 1 minute.

5. Add in the cooked vegetables and cook for about 2-3 minutes.

6. Serve hot.

Vegetarian Burgers

Servings: 4

Preparation time: 15 minutes

Cooking time: 16 minutes

Ingredients:

- 1-pound of firm tofu, drained, pressed, and crumbled
- ¾ cup of rolled oats
- ¼ cup of flaxseeds
- 2 cups of frozen spinach, thawed
- 1 medium onion, chopped finely
- 4 garlic cloves, minced
- 1 teaspoon of ground cumin
- 1 teaspoon of red pepper flakes, crushed
- Sea salt and freshly ground black pepper, to taste
- 2 tablespoons of olive oil
- 6 cups of fresh salad greens

Instructions:

1. In a large bowl, add all the Ingredients except oil and salad greens and blend until well combined.

2. Put aside for about 10 minutes.

3. Make desired size patties from the mixture.

4. In a nonstick frying pan, heat the oil over medium heat and cook the patties for 6-8 minutes per side.

5. Serve these patties alongside the salad greens.

Cauliflower with Peas

Servings: 4

Preparation time: 15 minutes

Cooking time: 15 minutes

Ingredients:

- 2 medium tomatoes, chopped
- ¼ cup of water
- 2 tablespoons of olive oil
- 3 garlic cloves, minced
- ½ tablespoon of fresh ginger, minced
- 1 teaspoon of ground cumin
- 2 teaspoons of ground coriander
- 1 teaspoon of cayenne pepper
- ¼ teaspoon of ground turmeric
- 2 cups of cauliflower, chopped
- 1 cup of fresh green peas, shelled
- Salt and ground black pepper, as required
- ½ cup of warm water

Instructions:

1. In a blender, add tomato and ¼ cup of water and pulse until a smooth puree form. Set aside.

2. In a large skillet, heat the oil over medium heat and sauté the garlic, ginger, green chilies and spices for about 1 minute.

3. Add the cauliflower, peas and tomato puree and cook, stirring for about 3-4 minutes.

4. Add the nice and cosy water and bring to a boil.

5. Reduce the heat to medium-low and cook, covered for about 8-10 minutes or until vegetables are done completely.

6. Serve hot.

Broccoli with Bell Peppers

Servings: 6

Preparation time: 15 minutes

Cooking time: 10 minutes

Ingredients:

- 2 tablespoons of olive oil
- 4 garlic cloves, minced
- 1 large white onion, sliced
- 2 cups of small broccoli florets
- 3 red bell peppers, seeded and sliced
- ¼ cup of low-sodium vegetable broth
- Salt and ground black pepper, as required

Instructions:

1. In a large skillet, heat the oil over medium heat and sauté the garlic for about 1 minute.
2. Add the onion, broccoli and bell peppers and fry for about 5 minutes.
3. Add the broth and fry for about 4 minutes more.
4. Serve hot.

Veggies Curry

Servings: 6

Preparation time: 25 minutes

Cooking time: 15 minutes

Ingredients:

- 1 tablespoon of olive oil
- 1 small yellow onion, chopped
- 1 teaspoon of fresh thyme, chopped
- 1 garlic clove, minced
- 8 ounces of fresh mushroom, sliced
- 1-pound Brussels sprouts
- 3 cups of fresh spinach
- Salt and ground black pepper, as required

Instructions:

1. In a large skillet, heat the oil over medium heat and sauté the onion for about 3-4 minutes.
2. Add the thyme and garlic and sauté for about 1 minute.
3. Add the mushrooms and cook for about 15 minutes or until caramelized.

4. Add the Brussels sprouts and cook for about 2-3 minutes.
5. Stir in the spinach and cook for about 3-4 minutes.
6. Stir in the salt and black pepper and take away from the heat.
7. Serve hot.

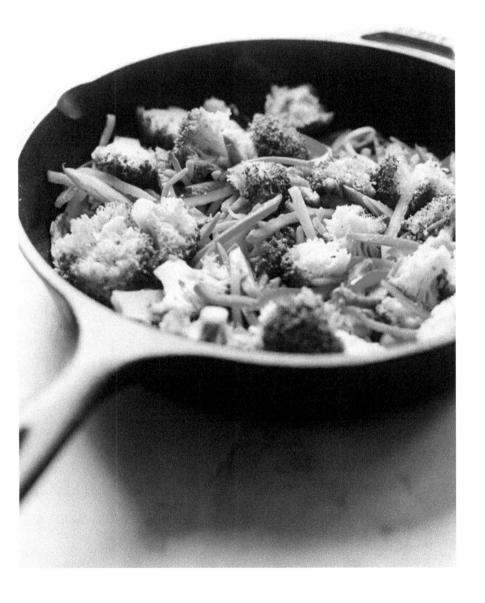

Veggies Combo

Servings: 4

Preparation time: 15 minutes

Cooking time: 10 minutes

Ingredients:

- 1 tablespoon of olive oil
- ½ cup of onion, sliced
- ½ cup of red bell pepper, seeded and julienned
- ½ cup of orange bell pepper, seeded and julienned
- 1½ cups of yellow squash, sliced
- 1½ cups of zucchini, sliced
- 1½ teaspoons of garlic, minced
- ¼ cup of water
- Salt and ground black pepper, as required

Instructions:

1. In a large skillet, heat the oil over medium-high heat and sauté the onion, bell peppers and squash for about 4-5 minutes.
2. Add the garlic and sauté for about 1 minute.

3. Add the remaining Ingredients and stir to mix.
4. Reduce the heat to medium and cook for about 3-4 minutes, stirring occasionally.
5. Serve hot.

Cauliflower with Peas

Servings: 4

Preparation time: 15 minutes

Cooking time: 15 minutes

Ingredients:

- 2 medium tomatoes, chopped
- ¼ cup of water
- 2 tablespoons of olive oil
- 3 garlic cloves, minced
- ½ tablespoon of fresh ginger, minced
- 1 teaspoon of ground cumin
- 2 teaspoons of ground coriander
- 1 teaspoon of cayenne pepper
- ¼ teaspoon of ground turmeric
- 2 cups of cauliflower, chopped
- 1 cup of fresh green peas, shelled
- Salt and ground black pepper, as required
- ½ cup of warm water

Instructions:

1. In a blender, add tomato and ¼ cup of water and pulse until a smooth puree form. Set aside.

2. In a large wok, heat oil over medium heat and sauté the garlic, ginger, green chilies and spices for about 1 minute.

3. Add the cauliflower, peas and tomato puree and cook, stirring for about 3-4 minutes.

4. Add the nice and cosy water and bring to a boil.

5. Adjust the heat to medium-low and cook, covered for about 8-10 minutes or until vegetables are done completely.

6. Serve hot.

Bok Choy & Mushroom Stir Fry

Servings: 4

Preparation time: 15 minutes

Cooking time: 10 minutes

Ingredients:

- 1-pound baby bok choy
- 4 teaspoons of olive oil
- 1 teaspoon of fresh ginger, minced
- 2 garlic cloves, chopped
- 5 ounces of fresh mushrooms, sliced
- 2 tablespoons of red wine
- 2 tablespoons of soy sauce
- Ground black pepper, as required

Instructions:

1. Trim bases of bok choy and separate outer leaves from stalks, leaving the littlest inner leaves attached.
2. In a large cast-iron wok, heat the oil over medium-high heat and sauté the ginger and garlic for about 1 minute.

3. Stir in the mushrooms and cook for about 4-5 minutes, stirring frequently.
4. Stir in the bok choy leaves and stalks and cook for about 1 minute, tossing with tongs.
5. Stir in the wine, soy and black pepper and cook for about 2-3 minutes, tossing occasionally.
6. Serve hot.

Orange Chicken

Servings: 6

Preparation time: 10 minutes

Cooking time: 20 minutes

Ingredients:

- 3 garlic cloves, minced
- ½ cup of fresh orange juice
- 1 tablespoon of apple cider vinegar
- 2 tablespoons of low-sodium soy sauce
- ¼ teaspoon of ground ginger
- ¼ teaspoon of ground cinnamon
- Freshly ground black pepper, to taste
- 2 pounds skinless, bone-in chicken thighs
- 1/3 cup of scallion, sliced

Instructions:

1. For marinating in a large bowl, mix together all Ingredients apart from chicken thighs and scallion.
2. Add the chicken thighs and coat with marinade generously.

3. Cover the bowl and refrigerate to marinate for about 4 hours.
4. Remove the chicken from the bowl, reserving marinade.
5. Heat a lightly greased large non-stick skillet over medium-high heat and cook the chicken thighs for about 5-6 minutes or till golden brown.
6. Flip the side and cook for about 4 minutes.
7. Stir in the reserved marinade and bring to a boil.
8. Reduce the heat to medium-low and cook, covered for about 6-8 minutes or until sauce becomes thick.
9. Stir in the scallion and take away from the heat.
10. Serve hot

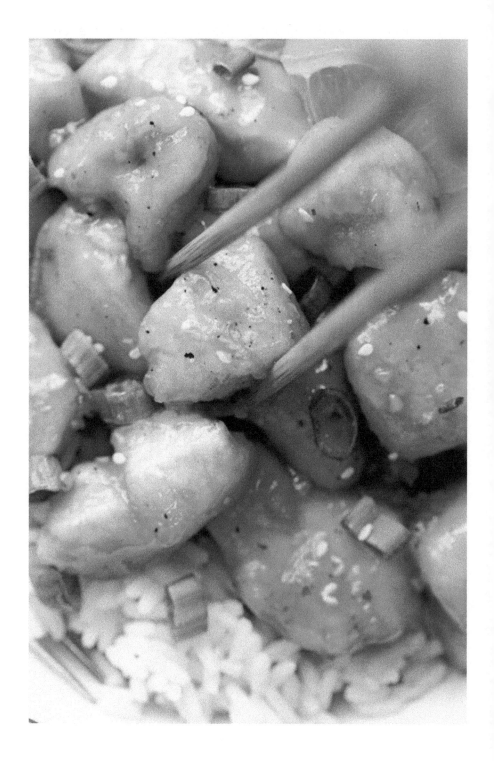

Chicken Breast with Asparagus

Servings: 5

Preparation time: 15 minutes

Cooking time: 16 minutes

Ingredients:

For Chicken:

- ¼ cup of extra-virgin olive oil
- ¼ cup of fresh lemon juice
- 2 tablespoons of maple syrup
- 1 garlic clove, minced
- Salt and ground black pepper, as required
- 5 (6-ounce of) boneless, skinless chicken breasts

For Asparagus:

- 1½ pounds of fresh asparagus
- 2 tablespoons of extra-virgin olive oil

Instructions:

1. For marinade: In a large bowl, add oil, lemon juice, Erythritol, garlic, salt, and black pepper, and beat until well combined.
2. In a large resealable bag, place the chicken and ¾ cup of marinade.
3. Seal the bag and shake to coat well.
4. Refrigerate overnight.
5. Cover the bowl of remaining marinade and refrigerate before serving.
6. Preheat the grill to medium heat. Grease the grill grate.
7. Remove the chicken from the bag and discard the marinade.
8. Place the chicken onto grill grate and grill, covered for about 5-8 minutes per side.
9. Meanwhile, in a pan of boiling water, arrange a steamer basket.
10. Place the asparagus in a steamer basket and steam, covered for about 5-7 minutes.
11. Drain the asparagus well and transfer into a bowl.
12. Add oil and toss to coat well.
13. Divide the chicken breasts and asparagus onto serving plates and serve.

Chicken with Zoodles

Servings: 4

Preparation time: 15 minutes

Cooking time: 18 minutes

Ingredients:

- 2 cups of zucchini, spiralized with Blade
- Salt, to taste
- 1½ pounds boneless, skinless chicken breasts
- Freshly ground black pepper, to taste
- 1 tablespoon of olive oil
- 1 cup of low-fat plain Greek yogurt
- ¼ cup of low-fat Parmesan cheese, shredded
- ½ cup of low-sodium chicken broth
- ½ teaspoon of Italian seasoning
- ½ teaspoon of garlic powder
- 1 cup of fresh spinach, chopped
- 3-6 slices of sun-dried tomatoes
- 1 tablespoon of garlic, chopped

Instructions:

1. Preheat your oven to 350 degrees F.
2. Line a large baking sheet with parchment paper.
3. Place the zucchini noodles and salt onto the prepared baking sheet and toss to coat well.
4. Arrange the zucchini noodles in a good layer and Bake for about 15 minutes.
5. Meanwhile, season the chicken breasts with salt and black pepper.
6. In a large skillet, heat the oil over medium-high heat and cook the chicken breasts for about 4-5 minutes per side or until cooked through.
7. With a slotted spoon, transfer the cooked chicken onto a plate and put aside.
8. In the same skillet, add the yogurt, Parmesan cheese, broth, Italian seasoning, and garlic powder and beat until well combined.
9. Place the skillet over medium-high heat and cook for about 2-3 minutes or until it starts to thicken, stirring continuously.
10. Stir in the spinach, sun-dried tomatoes, and garlic and cook for about 2-3 minutes.
11. Add the chicken breasts and cook for about 1-2 minutes.
12. Divide the zucchini noodles onto serving plates and top each with chicken mixture.
13. Serve immediately.

Chicken with Yellow Squash

Servings: 6

Preparation time: 15 minutes

Cooking time: 17 minutes

Ingredients:

- 2 tablespoons of olive oil, divided
- 1½ pounds skinless, boneless chicken breasts, cut into bite-sized pieces
- Salt and freshly ground black pepper, to taste
- 2 garlic cloves, minced
- 1½ pounds yellow squash, sliced
- 2 tablespoons of fresh lemon juice
- 1 teaspoon of fresh lemon zest, grated finely
- 2 tablespoons of fresh parsley, minced

Instructions:

1. In a large skillet, heat 1 tablespoon of oil over medium heat and fry chicken for about 6-8 minutes or until golden brown from all sides.
2. Transfer the chicken onto a plate.

3. In the same skillet, heat remaining oil over medium heat and sauté garlic for about 1 minute.
4. Add the squash slices and cook for about 5-6 minutes,
5. Stir in the chicken and cook for about 2 minutes.
6. Stir in the lemon juice, zest, and parsley and take away from heat.
7. Serve hot.

Chicken with Bell Peppers

Servings: 6

Preparation time: 15 minutes

Cooking time: 20 minutes

Ingredients:

- 3 tablespoons of olive oil, divided
- 1 yellow bell pepper, seeded and sliced
- 1 red bell pepper, seeded and sliced
- 1 green bell pepper, seeded and sliced
- 1 medium onion, sliced
- 1-pound boneless, skinless chicken breasts, sliced thinly1 teaspoon of dried oregano, crushed
- ¼ teaspoon of garlic powder
- ¼ teaspoon of ground cumin
- Salt and freshly ground black pepper, to taste
- ¼ cup of low-sodium chicken broth

Instructions:

1. In a skillet, heat 1 tablespoon of oil over medium-high heat and cook the bell peppers and onion slices for about 4-5 minutes.

2. With a slotted spoon, transfer the peppers mixture onto a plate.

3. In the same skillet, heat the remaining oil over medium-high heat and cook the chicken for about 8 minutes, stirring frequently.

4. Stir in the thyme, spices, salt, black pepper, and broth, and bring to a boil.

5. Add the peppers mixture and stir to mix.

6. Reduce the heat to medium and cook for about 3-5 minutes or until all the liquid is absorbed, stirring occasionally.

7. Serve immediately.

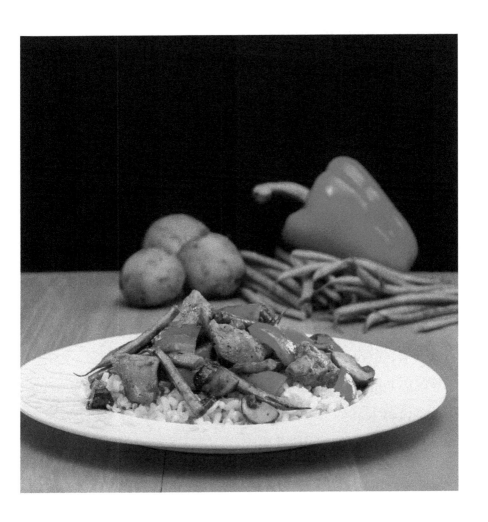

Chicken with Mushrooms

Servings: 4

Preparation time: 15 minutes

Cooking time: 20 minutes

Ingredients:

- 2 tablespoons of almond flour
- Salt and freshly ground black pepper, to taste
- 4 (4-ounce of) skinless, boneless chicken breasts
- 2 tablespoons of olive oil
- 6 garlic cloves, chopped
- ¾ pound fresh mushrooms, sliced
- ¾ cup of low-sodium chicken broth
- ¼ cup of balsamic vinegar
- 1 bay leaf
- ¼ teaspoon of dried thyme

Instructions:

1. In a bowl, mix together the flour, salt, and black pepper.
2. Coat the chicken breasts with flour mixture evenly.

3. In a skillet, heat the vegetable oil over medium-high heat and fry chicken for about 3 minutes.

4. Add the garlic and flip the chicken breasts.

5. Spread mushrooms over chicken and cook for about 3 minutes, shaking the skillet frequently.

6. Add the broth, vinegar, herb, and thyme and stir to mix.

7. Reduce the heat to medium-low and simmer, covered for about 10 minutes, flipping chicken occasionally.

8. With a slotted spoon, transfer the chicken onto a warm serving platter and with a bit of foil, cover to stay warm.

9. Place the pan of sauce over medium-high heat and cook, uncovered for about 7 minutes.

10. Remove the pan from heat and discard the herb.

11. Place sauce over chicken and serve hot.

Chicken with Broccoli

Servings: 4

Preparation time: 15 minutes

Cooking time: 22 minutes

Ingredients:

- 2 tablespoons of olive oil, divided
- 4 (4-ounce of) boneless, skinless chicken breasts, cut into small pieces
- Salt and freshly ground black pepper, to taste
- 1 onion, chopped finely
- 1 teaspoon of fresh ginger, grated
- 1 teaspoon of garlic, minced
- 1 cup of broccoli florets
- 1½ cups of fresh mushrooms, sliced
- 8 ounces of low-sodium chicken broth

Instructions:

1. In a large skillet, heat 1 tablespoon of oil over medium-high heat and fry the chicken pieces, salt, and black pepper for about 4-5 minutes or until golden brown.

2. With a slotted spoon, transfer the chicken onto a plate.

3. In the same skillet, heat the remaining oil over medium-high heat and sauté the onion, ginger, and garlic for about 4-5 minutes.

4. Add in mushrooms and cook for about 4-5 minutes, stirring frequently.

5. Add the broccoli and fry for about 3 minutes.

6. Add the cooked chicken and broth and fry for about 3-5 minutes

7. Add in the salt and black pepper and take away from the heat.

8. Serve hot.

Chicken & Veggies Stir Fry

Servings: 6

Preparation time: 15 minutes

Cooking time: 15 minutes

Ingredients:

- 2 tablespoons of fresh lime juice
- 2 tablespoons of fish sauce
- 1½ teaspoons of arrowroot starch
- 4 teaspoons of olive oil, divided
- 1-pound skinless, boneless chicken tenders, cubed
- 1 teaspoon of fresh ginger, minced
- 2 garlic cloves, minced
- ¾ teaspoon of red pepper flakes, crushed
- ¼ cup of water
- 4 cups of broccoli, cut into bite-sized pieces
- 3 cup of red bell pepper, seeded and sliced
- ¼ cup of pine nuts

Instructions:

1. In a bowl, add lemon juice, fish sauce, and arrowroot starch and blend until well combined. Set aside.
2. In a large non-stick sauté pan, heat 2 teaspoons of oil over high heat and cook chicken for about 6-8 minutes, stirring frequently.
3. Transfer the chicken into a bowl and put it aside.
1. 4 In an equivalent sauté pan, heat remaining oil over medium heat and sauté ginger, garlic, and red pepper
2. Flakes for about 1 minute.
3. 5 Add water, broccoli, and bell pepper and fry for about 2-3 minutes.
4. 6. Stir in chicken and juice mixture and cook for about 2-3 minutes.
8. Stir in pine nuts and immediately remove from heat.
9. Serve hot.

Chicken & Broccoli Bake

Servings: 6

Preparation time: 15 minutes

Cooking time: 24 minutes

Ingredients:

- Olive oil cooking spray
- 6 (6-ounce of) skinless, boneless chicken thighs
- 3 broccoli heads, cut into florets
- 4 garlic cloves, minced
- ¼ cup of extra-virgin olive oil
- 1 teaspoon of dried oregano, crushed
- 1 teaspoon of dried rosemary, crushed
- Salt and freshly ground black pepper, to taste

Instructions:

1. Preheat your oven to 375 degrees F.
2. Grease a large baking dish with cooking spray.
3. In a large bowl, add all the Ingredients and toss to coat well.

4. At the bottom of the prepared baking dish, arrange the broccoli florets and top with chicken breasts in a single layer.
5. Bake for about 45 minutes.
6. Serve hot.

Cheesy Chicken & Spinach

Servings: 4

Preparation time: 15 minutes

Cooking time: 20 minutes

Ingredients:

- 2 tablespoons of olive oil, divided
- 4 (4-ounce of) boneless, skinless chicken thighs
- Salt and ground black pepper, as required
- 2 garlic cloves, minced
- 1 jalapeño pepper, chopped
- 10-ounce of frozen spinach, thawed
- 1/3 cup of low-fat Parmesan cheese, shredded

Instructions:

1. In a large skillet, heat 1 tablespoon of the oil over medium-high heat and cook the chicken with salt and black pepper for about 5-6 minutes per side.
2. Transfer the chicken into a bowl.
3. In the same skillet, heat the remaining oil over medium-low heat and sauté the garlic for about 1 minute.

4. Add the spinach and cook for about 1 minute.

5. Add the cheese, salt, and black pepper and stir to mix.

1. 6 Spread the spinach mixture in the bottom of the skillet evenly.

2. 7 Place chicken over spinach in a single layer.

3. 8 Immediately adjust the heat to low and cook, covered for about 5 minutes.

4. 9 Serve hot.

Chicken & Cauliflower Curry

Servings: 6

Preparation time: 15 minutes

Cooking time: 20 minutes

Ingredients:

- ¼ cup of olive oil
- 3 garlic cloves, minced
- 2 tablespoons of curry powder
- 1½ pounds skinless, boneless chicken thighs, cut into bite-sized pieces
- Salt and ground black pepper, as required
- 1-pound cauliflower, cut into small pieces
- 1 green bell pepper, seeded and chopped
- 14 ounces of unsweetened coconut milk
- ¼ cup of fresh parsley, chopped

Instructions:

1. In a large skillet, heat the oil over medium heat and sauté the garlic and chili powder for about 1 minute.

2. Add the chicken, salt, and black pepper and cook for about 5-6 minutes, stirring frequently.
3. With a slotted spoon, transfer the chicken onto a plate.
4. In the skillet, add the cauliflower and bell pepper and cook for about 2-3 minutes.
5. Add the coconut milk and simmer for about 5-7 minutes.
6. Stir in the cooked chicken, salt, and black pepper, and cook for about 2-3 minutes.
7. Serve hot with the garnishing of parsley.

Chicken & Veggies Casserole

Servings: 4

Preparation time: 15 minutes

Cooking time: 25 minutes

Ingredients:

- 1 tablespoon of olive oil
- 1 small onion, chopped
- 1 pepperoni pepper, seeded and sliced thinly
- ½ of red bell pepper, seeded and sliced thinly
- 2 teaspoons of garlic, minced
- 1 cup of fresh spinach, trimmed and chopped
- ½ teaspoon of dried oregano
- Salt and freshly ground black pepper, to taste
- 4 (5-ounce of) skinless, boneless chicken breasts, butterflied and pounded

Instructions:

1. Preheat your oven to 350 degrees F.
2. Line a baking sheet with parchment paper.

3. In a saucepan, heat the vegetable oil over medium heat and sauté onion and both peppers for about 1 minute.

4. Add the garlic and spinach and cook for about 2-3 minutes or until just wilted.

5. Stir in oregano, salt, and black pepper, and take away the saucepan from heat.

6. Place the chicken mixture into the center of every butterflied chicken breast.

7. Fold each chicken breast over filling to form a touch pocket and secure with toothpicks.

8. Arrange the chicken breasts onto the prepared baking sheet.

9. Bake for about 18-20 minutes.

10. Serve hot.

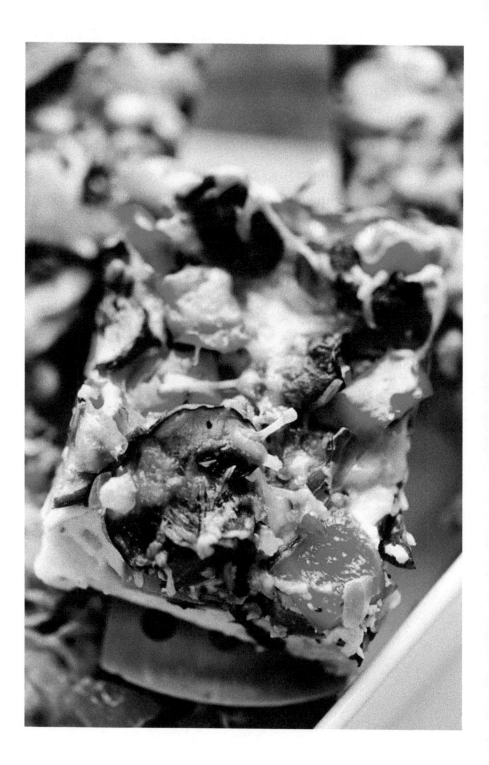

Chicken & Green Veggies Curry

Servings: 4

Preparation time: 15 minutes

Cooking time: 30 minutes

Ingredients:

- 1-pound skinless, boneless chicken breasts, cubed
- 1 tablespoon of olive oil
- 2 tablespoons of green curry paste
- 1 cup of unsweetened coconut milk
- 1 cup of low-sodium chicken broth
- 1 cup of asparagus spears, trimmed
- 1 cup of green beans, trimmed
- Salt and ground black pepper, as required
- ¼ cup of fresh cilantro leaves, chopped

Instructions:

1. In a skillet, heat oil over medium heat and sauté the curry paste for about 1-2 minutes.
2. Add the chicken and cook for about 8-10 minutes.
3. Add coconut milk and broth and bring to a boil.

4. Reduce the heat low and cook for about 8-10 minutes.

5. Add asparagus, green beans, salt, black pepper and cook for about 4-5 minutes or until desired doneness.

6. Serve hot.

Turkey & Avocado Lettuce Wraps

Servings: 2

Preparation time: 15 minutes

Cooking time: 13 minutes

Ingredients:

- 4 ounces of lean ground turkey
- ¼ cup of white onion, minced
- 2 tablespoons of sugar-free tomato sauce
- 1/8 teaspoon of ground cumin
- Freshly ground black pepper, to taste
- 2 teaspoons of extra-virgin olive oil
- 1 cup of tomato, chopped
- ½ cup of avocado, peeled, pitted, and chopped
- 1 tablespoon of fresh cilantro, chopped
- 4 large butternut lettuce leaves

Instructions:

1. 1 In a bowl, add the turkey, onion, pasta sauce, cumin, and black pepper and blend until well combined.

2. 2 In a large skillet, heat the oil over medium heat and cook the turkey mixture for about 8-10 minutes.

3. 3 Add the tomato and stir to mix.

4. 4 Immediately reduce the heat to low and cook for about 2-3 minutes.

5. Remove from the heat and put aside to chill.

6. Arrange the lettuce leaves onto serving plates.

7. Place the turkey mixture over each lettuce leaf evenly and top with avocado pieces.

8. Garnish with cilantro and serve immediately.

Turkey Burgers

Servings: 2

Preparation time: 15 minutes

Cooking time: 6 minutes

Ingredients:

For Burgers:

- 8 ounces of ground turkey
- Salt and ground black pepper, as required
- 1 ounce of part-skim Mozzarella cheese, cubed
- 1 tablespoon of olive oil

For Serving:

- 4 cups of fresh baby spinach
- 1 small cucumber, chopped

Instructions:

1. In a bowl, add the meat, salt, and black pepper and blend until well combined.
2. Make 2 equal-sized patties from the mixture.

3. Place mozzarella cues over each patty, and with your finger, press inside.
4. In a skillet, heat oil over medium heat and cook the patties for about 2-3 minutes per side.
5. Serve immediately alongside the spinach and cucumber.

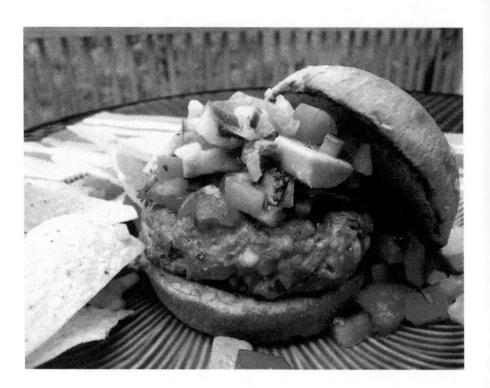

Turkey, Apple & Veggies Burgers

Servings: 4

Preparation time: 20 minutes

Cooking time: 12 minutes

Ingredients:

For Burgers:

- 12 ounces of lean ground turkey
- ½ of apple, peeled, cored, and grated
- ½ of red bell pepper, seeded and chopped finely
- ¼ cup of red onion, minced
- 2 small garlic cloves, minced
- 1 tablespoon of fresh ginger, minced
- 2½ tablespoons of fresh cilantro, chopped
- 2 tablespoons of curry paste1 teaspoon of ground cumin
- 1 teaspoon of olive oil

For Serving:

- 6 cups of fresh baby spinach

Instructions:

1. Preheat the grill to medium heat. Grease the grill grate.
2. For Burgers: in a large bowl, add all the Ingredients apart from oil and blend until well combined.
3. Make 4 equal-sized burgers from the mixture.
4. Brush the burgers with vegetable oil evenly.
5. Place the burgers onto the grill and cook for about 5-6 minutes per side. 6. Divide the baby spinach onto serving plates and top each with 1 burger.
6. Serve immediately.

Turkey Stuffed Zucchini

Servings: 8

Preparation time: 15 minutes

Cooking time: 31 minutes

Ingredients:

- 4 medium zucchinis
- 1-pound lean ground turkey breast
- ½ cup of white onion, chopped
- ½ pound fresh mushrooms, sliced
- 1 large tomato, chopped
- 1 egg, beaten
- ¾ cup of sugar-free spaghetti sauce
- ¼ cup of seasoned whole wheat bread crumbs
- Freshly ground black pepper, to taste
- 1 cup of low-fat mozzarella cheese, shredded

Instructions:

1. Preheat your oven to 350 degrees F.
2. Cut each zucchini in half lengthwise.

3. With a pointy knife, cut a skinny slice from the rock bottom of every zucchini to permit zucchini to take a seat flat.

4. With a little spoon, scoop out the pulp from each zucchini half, leaving ¼-inch shells.

5. Transfer the zucchini pulp into a large bowl and put it aside.

6. Arrange the zucchini shells into an ungreased microwave-safe baking dish.

7. Cover the baking dish and microwave on High for about 3 minutes.

8. Drain the water from the microwave and put it aside.

9. Heat a large non-stick skillet over medium heat and cook the bottom turkey and onion for about 6-8 minutes or until meat is no longer pink.

10. Drain the grease completely.

11. Remove from the heat.

12. In the bowl of zucchini pulp, add the cooked turkey, mushrooms, tomato, egg, spaghetti sauce, black pepper, and ½ cup of the cheese and blend until well combined.

13. Place about ¼ cup of the turkey mixture into each zucchini shell and sprinkle with the remaining cheese.

14. Bake for about 20 minutes or until the top becomes golden brown.

15. Serve hot.

Turkey Stuffed Acorn Squash

Servings: 4

Preparation time: 15 minutes

Cooking time: 50 minutes

Ingredients:

- 2 acorn squash, halved and seeded 1-pound lean ground turkey breast
- 1 cup of red onion, chopped
- 1 cup of celery stalk, chopped
- 1 cup of fresh button mushrooms, sliced
- 8 ounces of sugar-free tomato sauce
- 1 teaspoon of dried oregano, crushed
- 1 teaspoon of dried basil, crushed
- Freshly ground black pepper, to taste
- 1 cup of low-fat Cheddar cheese, shredded

Instructions:

1. Preheat your oven to 350 degrees F.
2. In the bottom of a microwave-safe glass baking dish, arrange the squash halves, cut side down.

3. Microwave on High for about 20 minutes or until almost tender.

4. Heat a large non-stick skillet over medium heat and cook the bottom turkey for about 4-5 minutes or until meat is no longer pink.

5. Drain the grease completely.

6. Add the onion and celery and cook for about 3-4 minutes.

7. Stir in the mushrooms and cook for about 2-3 minutes more.

8. Stir in the spaghetti sauce, dried herbs, and black pepper and take away from the heat.

9. Spoon the turkey mixture into each squash half.

10. Cover the baking dish and bake for about 15 minutes.

11. Uncover the baking dish and sprinkle each squash half with cheddar.

12. Bake uncovered for about 3-5 minutes or until the cheese becomes bubbly.

13. Serve hot.

Turkey & Spinach Meatballs

Servings: 4

Preparation time: 20 minutes

Cooking time: 15 minutes

Ingredients:

For Meatballs:

- 1-pound lean ground turkey
- 1 cup of frozen chopped spinach, thawed and squeezed
- ½ cup of feta cheese, crumbled
- ½ teaspoon of dried oregano
- Salt and ground black pepper, as required
- 2 tablespoons of olive oil

For Salad:

- 4 cups of lettuce, torn
- 2 large tomatoes, chopped
- 1 cup of onion, sliced
- 2 tablespoons of olive oil
- Salt and ground black pepper, as required

Instructions:

1. For meatballs: place all Ingredients apart from oil in a bowl and blend until well combined.
2. Make 12 equal-sized meatballs from the mixture.
3. Heat the vegetable oil in a large non-stick skillet over medium heat and cook the meatballs for about 10-15 minutes or until done completely, flipping occasionally.
4. With a slotted spoon, transfer the meatballs onto a plate.
5. Meanwhile, For Salad: In a large salad bowl, add all Ingredients and toss to coat well.
6. Divide meatballs and salad onto serving plates and serve.

Turkey Meatballs Kabobs

Servings: 4

Preparation time: 15 minutes

Cooking time: 14 minutes

Ingredients:

- 1 yellow onion, chopped roughly
- ½ cup of lemongrass, chopped roughly
- 2 garlic cloves, chopped roughly
- 1½ pounds of lean ground turkey
- 1 teaspoon of sesame oil
- ½ tablespoons of low-sodium soy sauce
- 1 tablespoon of arrowroot starch
- 1/8 teaspoon of powdered stevia
- Salt and ground black pepper, as required
- 6 cups of fresh baby spinach

Instructions:

1. Preheat the grill to medium-high heat.
2. Grease the grill grate.

3. In a food processor, add the onion, lemongrass, and garlic and pulse until chopped finely.

4. Transfer the onion mixture into a large bowl.

5. Add the remaining Ingredients apart from spinach and blend until well combined.

6. Make 12 equal-sized balls from the meat mixture.

7. Thread the balls onto the presoaked wooden skewers.

8. Place the skewers onto the grill and cook for about 6-7 minutes per side.

9. Serve hot alongside the spinach.

Turkey with Peas

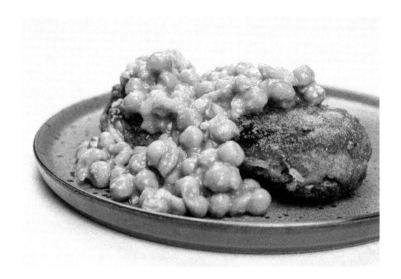

Servings: 6

Preparation time: 15 minutes

Cooking time: 40 minutes

Ingredients:

- 2 tablespoons of extra virgin olive oil
- 1-pound lean ground turkey
- 1 large white onion, chopped finely
- 2 garlic cloves, minced
- ½ tablespoon of fresh ginger, minced
- 1 teaspoon of ground coriander
- 1 teaspoon of ground cumin

- ¼ teaspoon of chili powder
- 2 medium tomatoes, seeded and chopped
- ½ cup of low-sodium chicken broth
- Salt and freshly ground black pepper, to taste
- 2 cups of fresh peas, shelled
- 2 tablespoons of fresh cilantro, chopped

Instructions:

1. In a large skillet, heat the oil over medium heat and cook the turkey for about 4-5 minutes or until browned completely.
2. With a slotted spoon, transfer the turkey into a large bowl.
3. In the same skillet, add the onion and sauté for about 4-6 minutes.
4. Add the garlic, ginger, coriander, cumin, and chili powder and sauté for about 1 minute.
5. Add the tomatoes and cook for about 2-3 minutes, crushing completely with the rear of the spoon.
6. Stir in the cooked turkey, broth, salt, and black pepper and bring to a boil.
7. Reduce the heat to medium-low and simmer, covered for about 8-10 minutes, stirring occasionally.
8. Stir in peas and cook for about 15-20 minutes.

9. Remove from the heat and serve hot with the garnishing of almonds and cilantro leaves.

Turkey & Veggie Casserole

Servings: 6

Preparation time: 15 minutes

Cooking time: 50 minutes

Ingredients:

- 2 medium zucchinis, sliced
- 2 medium tomatoes, sliced
- ¾ pound ground turkey
- 1 large yellow onion, chopped
- 2 garlic cloves, minced
- 1 cup of sugar-free tomato sauce
- ½ cup of low-fat cheddar cheese, shredded
- 2 cups of cottage cheese, shredded
- 1 egg yolk
- 1 tablespoon of fresh rosemary, minced
- Salt and ground black pepper, as required

Instructions:

1. Preheat your oven to 500 degrees F.
2. Grease a large roasting pan
3. Arrange zucchini and tomato slices into the prepared roasting pan and spray with some cooking spray.
4. Roast for about 10-12 minutes.
5. Remove from oven and put aside.
6. Now, preheat your oven to 350 degrees F.
7. Meanwhile, heat a nonstick skillet over medium-high heat and cook the turkey for about 4-5 minutes or until browned.
8. Add the onion and garlic and sauté for about 4-5 minutes.
9. Stir in spaghetti sauce and cook for about 2-3 minutes.
10. Remove from the heat and place the turkey mixture into a 13x9-inch shallow baking dish.
11. In a bowl, add the remaining Ingredients and blend until well combined.
12. Place the roasted vegetables over the turkey mixture, followed by the cheese mixture evenly.
13. Bake for about 35 minutes.
14. Remove from the oven and put aside for about 5-10 minutes.
15. Cut into equal-sized 8 wedges and serve.

Turkey Chili

Servings: 8

Preparation time: 15 minutes

Cooking time: 2¼ hours

Ingredients:

- 2 tablespoons of olive oil
- 1 small yellow onion, chopped
- 1 green bell pepper, seeded and chopped
- 4 garlic cloves, minced
- 1 jalapeño pepper, chopped
- 1 teaspoon of dried thyme, crushed
- 2 tablespoons of red chili powder
- 1 tablespoon of ground cumin
- 2 pounds lean ground turkey
- 2 cups of fresh tomatoes, chopped finely
- 2 ounces of sugar-free tomato paste
- 2 cups of homemade low-sodium chicken broth
- 1 cup of water
- Salt and ground black pepper, as required

Instructions:

1. In a large Dutch oven, heat oil over medium heat and sauté the onion and bell pepper for about 5-7 minutes.
2. Add the garlic, jalapeno, thyme, and spices and sauté for about 1 minute.
3. Add the turkey and cook for about 4-5 minutes.
4. Stir in the tomatoes, ingredient, and cacao powder and cook for about 2 minutes.
5. Add in the broth and water and bring to a boil.
6. Now, reduce the heat to low and simmer, covered for about 2 hours.
7. Add in salt and black pepper and take away from the heat.
8. Serve hot.

Turkey & Veggie Casserole

Servings: 6

Preparation time: 20 minutes

Cooking time: 1 hour

Ingredients:

- 2 medium zucchinis, sliced
- 2 medium tomatoes, sliced
- Olive oil cooking spray
- ¾ pound of ground turkey
- 1 large yellow onion, chopped
- 2 garlic cloves, minced
- 1 cup of sugar-free tomato sauce
- ½ cup of low-fat cheddar cheese, shredded
- 2 cups of cottage cheese, shredded
- 1 egg yolk
- 1 tablespoon of fresh rosemary, minced
- Salt and ground black pepper, as required

Instructions:

1. Preheat your oven to 500 degrees F.

2. Grease a large roasting pan.

3. Arrange zucchini and tomato slices into the prepared roasting pan and spray with some cooking spray.

4. Roast for about 10-12 minutes.

5. Remove from oven and put aside.

6. Now, preheat your oven to 350 degrees F.

7. Meanwhile, heat a non-stick skillet over medium-high heat and cook the turkey for about 4-5 minutes or until brown.

8. Add the onion and garlic and sauté for about 4-5 minutes.

9. Stir in spaghetti sauce and cook for about 2-3 minutes.

10. Remove from the heat and place the turkey mixture into a 13x9-inch shallow baking dish.

11. In a bowl, add the remaining Ingredients and blend until well combined.

12. Place the roasted vegetables over the turkey mixture, followed by the cheese mixture evenly.

13. Bake for about 35 minutes.

14. Remove from the oven and put aside for about 5-10 minutes.

15. Divide into desired sized pieces and serve.

Beef Lettuce Wraps

Servings: 2

Preparation time: 15 minutes

Cooking time: 13 minutes

Ingredients:

- 2 tablespoons of white onion, chopped
- 5 ounces of lean ground beef
- 2 tablespoons of light thousand island dressing
- 1/8 teaspoon of white vinegar
- 1/8 teaspoon of onion powder
- 4 lettuce leaves
- 2 tablespoons of low-fat cheddar cheese, shredded
- 1 small cucumber, julienned

Instructions:

1. Heat a little, lightly greased skillet over medium-high heat, and sauté the onion for about 2-3 minutes.
2. Add the meat and cook for about 8-10 minutes or until cooked through.
3. Remove from the heat and put aside.

4. In a bowl, add the dressing, vinegar, and onion powder and blend well.

5. Arrange the lettuce leaves onto serving plates.

6. Place beef mixture over each lettuce leaf, followed by the cheese and cucumber.

7. Drizzle with sauce and serve.

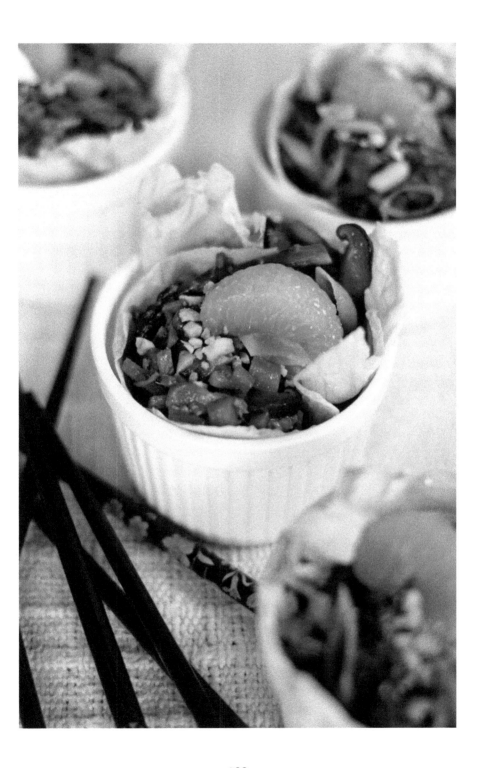

Lightning Source UK Ltd.
Milton Keynes UK
UKHW020807180621
385732UK00001B/88